W9-AUP-483

STYLISH SETTINGS

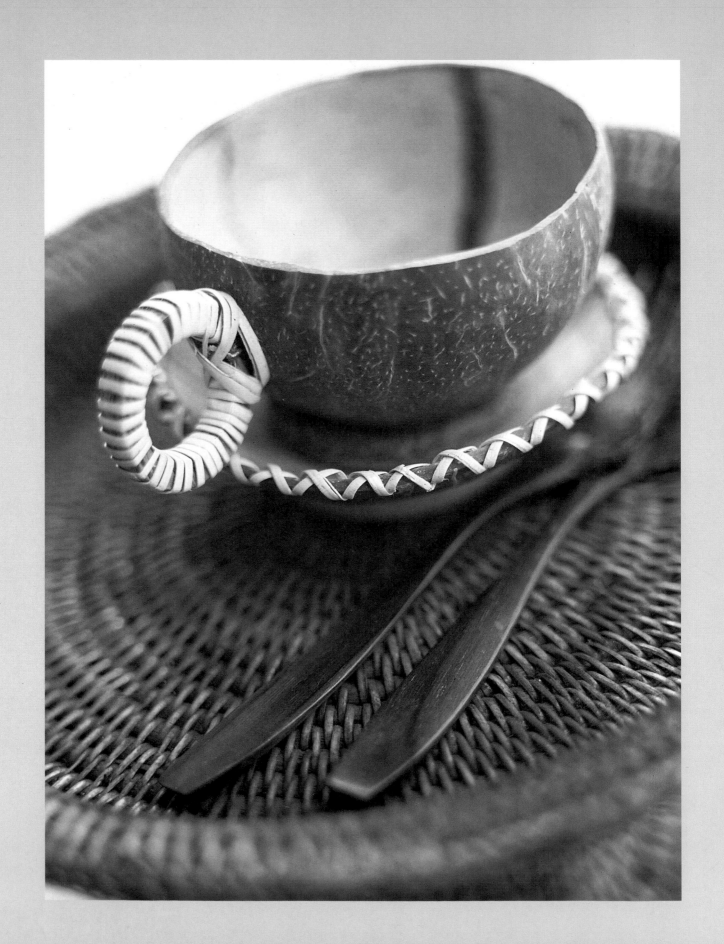

STYLISH SETTINGS

THE ART
OF CREATING
A BEAUTIFUL
TABLE

MARGARET CASELTON

WEIDENFELD
& NICOLSON
LONDON

FOR EMILY, WITH LOVE

First published in 1996 by
George Weidenfeld & Nicolson Limited
The Orion Publishing Group
Orion House
5 Upper St. Martin's Lane
London WC2H 9EA

Text © Margaret Caselton 1996
Margaret Caselton has asserted her right
to be identified as the Author of this
Work.

All rights reserved. No part of this
publication may be reproduced, stored in
a retrieval system, or transmitted in any
form or by any means, electronic,
mechanical or otherwise, without prior
permission of the copyright holder.

British Library Cataloguing-in-
Publication Data
A catalogue record for this book is
available from the British Library.

ISBN 0-297-83548-3

Designed by Nigel Soper

CONTENTS

6
INTRODUCTION

8
BLUE AND WHITE

28
CONTEMPORARY
CLASSICS

50
INFLUENCES FROM AFAR

70
ALFRESCO

84
SPECIAL OCCASIONS

114
FLORIBUNDA

128
APPENDIX & INDEX

INTRODUCTION

I have always loved tabletop things: china, knives, forks, spoons, and glasses. Yet my china cupboard boasts only one complete set of matching pieces — and those I inherited from my mother. I collect cutlery from street markets and buy innovative and unusual pieces from crafts galleries. My glass cupboard is a hodgepodge of different styles, from inexpensive but classic wineglasses — what the Victorians discreetly but accurately termed elegant economy — to a few pieces of Lalique, mingled in with colored glassware and Moroccan mint tea glasses. Wherever I go I come back with something for the table.

Table setting for me is not about abiding by strict rules of etiquette. It is about creating your own still life — having fun with a dash of color here, mixing crockery patterns there, and deciding on which tablecloth provides the best background color.

My method is to select several pieces and experiment with one place setting, then I add another element or change the color of a glass, place a flower, and stand back and squint as if at a painting.

I adore flowers and for me they are the crowning glory of the setting. They are good friends — there to help you out. They complete the effect, lend softness of texture and natural color and form. It is essential to work flowers in tandem with the menu to avoid unappetizing collisions of color.

I have tried to incorporate a visual example of plain white china into most settings. White china is an ideal basic set, as it can be used very effectively to complement or contrast with any color, even gold and silver for a grand occasion.

Essentially this is a collection of ideas, a coloring book of themes and collages, and a few menu suggestions. I have also included a section on international table settings for reference, but they are not intended as the last word. There are several excellent books on modern etiquette available with much more detailed advice.

The ideas presented in this book are meant to encourage experimentation and boldness with color combinations, and to inspire confidence in developing a personal style. The important thing is not to worry about overdoing it — a bit of exuberance adds to the jollity of the occasion.

Bon appétit and have fun.

BLUE AND WHITE

Blue and white china has been popular for more than 400 years. It originated in China, where cobalt blue was painted onto porcelain as decoration before glazing. Imported by the East India companies into Europe, "china" became so established in Holland that it is known as Delft, after the Dutch town that became the major European center for its production. Important Staffordshire potteries in England, particularly Spode, manufactured transfer-printed designs, making blue and white china in a myriad of patterns – many of them Chinese – available to everyone. Odd pieces of these sets still exist and look very effective when grouped together. Such pieces may be easily picked up at antique fairs and markets, and larger sets might be found at auction houses. Collecting is an interesting hobby and valuable pieces sometimes turn up unexpectedly. Blue and white patterns are still in production, such as the traditional Willow, Spode's Blue Italian (which has been in continuous production since 1816), Geranium, Tower pattern, Asiatic Pheasant, and the elegant Blue Flowers by Royal Copenhagen. A good idea is to mix your collected blue and white china and, depending on the occasion, set it against a white or patterned blue cloth with a bunch of seasonal flowers.

FRENCH BISTRO

This is a friendly, informal setting for lunch which is simple and fresh. Your choice of table setting will convey the mood of the occasion before the guests even sit down. A cheerful café style is achieved with a basic theme of blues and white, juxtaposed with checks and stripes. China and flatware are simple, utilitarian, and dishwasher-proof. Each setting is contained and uncluttered. The key to simplicity is a carefully considered use of color, pattern, and texture, built layer upon layer. Complete the look with equally simple accessories and details such as the checked napkin used as a focal point and a salad bowl potted with small daisies.

LEFT *Informal table settings call for informal flowers such as daisies – in a dainty bunch or a generous bowl.*

A pretty Victorian silver cruet set provides the necessary condiments and spices. Items you may have stored away in cupboards can be put to good use, serving a visual and functional purpose. This little set could be used equally well at a formal dinner, and here it injects a touch of elegance which offsets the "chunky" tableware.

A careful combination of detail sets the mood. The basic theme of blue and white creates a lively, informal atmosphere when set against a background of blue table linen in checks and stripes. An informal lunch means light but nourishing food. Here broiled goat cheese on bruschetta is served on a bed of lamb's lettuce and chopped walnuts, dressed with extra virgin olive oil.

Café-style china and glasses need to be offset by lighter elements such as country flowers.

Saturation and density of color can be achieved by the

juxtaposition of different tones and patterns. Bring together

mismatched linen, kitchen china, flatware, glasses – all in the

chosen base colors – and place them together. A variety of napkins

– such as one striped, one checked, one plain – looks cheerful.

Informal settings are often

used in bistros. The knife

and fork are placed

together and set on a

napkin to one side of the

plate or on the plate.

Create a country atmosphere by using a homely container for flowers. Milk pitchers, enamel pitchers, or even jam jars filled with buttercups, dandelions, or common meadow flowers look charming. (Make sure they are plentiful and not a protected species before you pick them.) Tablecloths should be equally simple and can be cotton gingham, striped, or plain. Start a collection or make them from colorful dress or upholstery fabrics.

LEFT *Bread can be placed directly on the table in French café style.*

ASIATIC PHEASANT

A collection of Asiatic Pheasant, which was first produced in Victorian times, forms the basis of a special late-spring setting. The blue and white theme is enhanced by the soft pink and green of the full-blown peonies. As the china is not a complete set, we introduced floral-decorated coffee cups to complement the peonies. Table linen is fresh, starched, and white, with subtle floral embroidery. The original Asiatic Pheasant had a soft blue pattern, and became fashionable in the 1840s. The popularity of the pattern led to its being reproduced in the 1980s, and these modern versions can still be found, although the blue glaze may be somewhat darker than that found on the originals.

RIGHT *Simple glassware is best for lunch. Embellished glassware may look fussy, but pale pink or pale blue glasses would be effective.*

LEFT *Set on the table are the elements of a late-spring lunch party setting. The color theme consists of pink, blue, and white.*

RIGHT *Detail of china and flatware for one setting, showing the Asiatic Pheasant pattern.*

RIGHT *Stacked plates – old and new – in the popular Asiatic Pheasant design. The soft blue glaze lends a delicacy that can be enhanced by the juxtaposition of other soft colors.*

The Asiatic Pheasant pattern has been popular since the 1840s, and old and new pieces may still be found. This collection has been put together over more than 20 years.

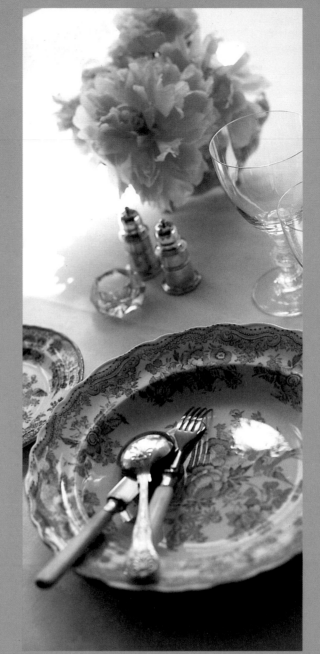

Attention to detail is important, including the harmony of the color scheme, the texture and design of the linen, and the style of the flatware.

FAR LEFT *Some of these napkins are new and some are from antique shows or flea markets. All of them would be suitable for use in this setting.*

LEFT *It is important to establish a balanced composition of items of different height on the table – flowers, glasses, salt cellar and pepper shaker in this case.*

Flowers bring the setting to life and add a softness of texture. Buy flowers such as peonies and roses two days before you need them and let them open out.

BELOW *An example of the revived Asiatic Pheasant patterned china, which is currently in production. The blue glaze may have a darker hue than original pieces.*

One simple place setting in Asiatic Pheasant. All items, whether old or new, are linked by the 19th-century pattern and style.

A subtle floral theme links several elements such as the table linen, coffee-cup pattern, and peonies. Such detail is not always immediately noticeable but supports the harmony of the whole.

HARLEQUIN
BLUE

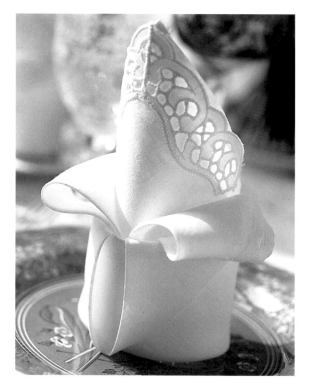

Spode blue-and-white-patterned plates from
the Georgian Plate Collection, with different
tones of blue underglaze and overlaying
patterns, make an attractive table display. The
blue-handled knives can easily be found at flea
markets or antique shows. The "bishop's miter"
napkin fold adds to the general embellishment;
folding instructions are on page 138.

LEFT *A detail of the china showing Spode's Botanical, which was introduced in 1826 in response to a growing interest in botany.*

ABOVE *Richly embellished hock and wine glasses echo the blue and white theme.*

A collection of old and new blue-and-white-patterned china is set out for a formal supper party on a summer's evening. On the table are two centerpieces for summer or winter: use both if you wish. If flowers are to be left on the table, they should be low so that guests can easily talk across the table. However, the generosity and height of this bunch creates a focus and a talking point. Flowers may also be cut to an equal length and one placed on each plate — some can last up to an hour in this way. Flowers brought by a guest could be used for this purpose. These would, of course, be removed before serving began.

RIGHT *A display of
the accessories used in
a blue and white
table setting.*

Use any blue and white dishes, a cake stand in white

china, blue- or white-handled knives – anything that

will enhance the theme. White embroidered table

linen and a pleasing bunch of white country flowers

and foliage bring life to the setting.

LEFT AND BELOW
*This stack of blue and
white plates was
collected over 10 years.
Red pears displayed on a
Royal Copenhagen cake
stand create a pleasing
centerpiece and add
height.*

*Many patterns of blue and white china have
been in continuous production since the early
1800s. For this reason they are easy to find and
it should not take long to build up a small
collection.*

CONTEMPORARY CLASSICS

There is such an enormous variety of tableware available to us, from so many parts of the world, that it is difficult sometimes to choose a service. Many contemporary examples will stand the test of time and become tomorrow's classics. A fine white dinner service will not date and looks effective on white table linen with simple flowers, or against a strong color. Most wedding china will be similar in style to our gold service (pages 30–31). The border color will differ, and can be taken as the theme. Notable also are Fornasetti's witty black and white and the colorful exuberance of Maryse Boxer's Rainbow china, left.

CLASSIC GOLD SERVICE

This elegant summer's evening setting for two or more uses a fine dinner service and crystal that are often included on wedding lists. Because it is simple and classic in design and style, the service can be used for different occasions. The key is the use of accessories to change the mood. Here a romantic setting is created by the unusual color of the full-blown roses and by keeping other colors warm, building upon the gold – the subtle edging of the glasses, the gold knot that decorates the flatware, the gold border of the napkins, and deep yellow beeswax candles.

ABOVE *Place a gold-topped salt and pepper shaker set at each place setting. Alternatively, one set can be shared between two guests.*

LEFT *The silver flatware features a subtle gold knot in keeping with the color scheme.*

CONTEMPORARY

CLASSICS

This setting is predominantly gold and white. Any glassware should be clear, and accessories should be chosen carefully to harmonize with the color scheme. The gold and crystal sparkling in the warm glow of candlelight make for a romantic setting and create a comfortable, intimate atmosphere. Decanters, although not always necessary, add to the sense of occasion. Little bonbonnières may be used to hold candy, and taller dishes to show off fruits such as pink grapes, cherries, or peaches — anything to augment the color scheme and textures. A finger bowl filled with rose water and floating rose petals may be put on the table during the dessert course. Such details add to the splendor and romance of the occasion, ensuring the evening is special from beginning to end. Beeswax candles, the color of soft

parchment, burn quickly. Keep supplies handy, as they will need replacing. Roses in an unusual lilac color were bought two days earlier so they would "blow." The rose theme is repeated in the napkin rings.

LEFT *The accessories used in this setting reflect the gold and white color scheme — the crystal clarity of the glassware, the color of the roses, even the candy in the bonbonnière with their gold wrappers.*

RIGHT *If the first course is soup, the elements of a place setting are dinner plate, entrée plate, soup bowl, and bread-and-butter plate; a red-wine glass and a white-wine glass; dinner knife and fork, dessert spoon and fork, and soup spoon; coffee cup, saucer, and coffee spoon; and, of course, a generously sized napkin.*

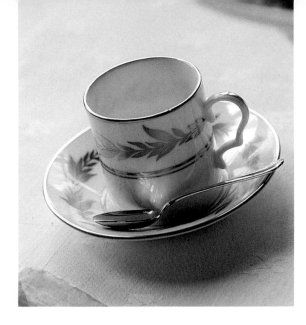

The combination of gold, crystal, and rich, full-blown roses create an opulent setting. The choice of color of roses can change the setting from pretty to richly romantic. Tight-budded white roses with the gold make a pretty setting, while rich, velvety, dark red Nicole roses are emphatically romantic.

LEFT *From beginning to end everything must be perfect – even the coffee cups.*

LEFT *A detail of the placement of flatware. The napkin is placed on top of the soup bowl. The white-wine glass is usually placed to the right of the red.*

ABOVE AND RIGHT *Remove the thorns and tie a moss-green velvet ribbon onto the stem of a rose. Fold the napkin into a slim cylinder-shape, and tie the ribbon around it.*

BLACK AND WHITE

The combination of black and white creates an air of formality and cosmopolitan living. The juxtaposition of such dramatic opposites creates a stunning table setting. Fornasetti's designs based on optical effects and architectural perspective provide a lively variation on a theme. Many of the designs work together to produce a fascinating interplay of visual effects – witty and elegant at the same time. Black and white work well with the injection of a single strong color such as gold. Here we have used Fornasetti plates and gold-rimmed glasses set upon upholstery fabric that works effectively as a tablecloth.

LEFT *Fornasetti plates and gold-rimmed glassware set upon fabric printed with a classical design.*

BELOW *A simple theme of black and white may be easily achieved with white plates, a black tablecloth, and silver accessories.*

LEFT *The sun was a favorite motif of Fornasetti and it works as a simple, elegant design on this dinner service. With the current trend for East-meets-West cuisine, chopsticks can be useful and decorative.*

BELOW *Imaginary architecture is another favorite Fornasetti theme. Here architectural forms provide a decorative border on a classic dinner service. On dinner plates a white center with a decorative rim is often preferred for food presentation.*

Gold and silver accessories, bringing luster and sparkle, are the perfect foil for the black and white in the Fornasetti table setting. Vases are simple and flowers neat and budded. The cloth – Renaissance Collage by the English team Timney Fowler – forms the perfect backdrop with its vivid shapes of color.

Left This wall plate with its classical design can also be used in the dinner service, especially against a cloth of roman coins on a black background.

Right Serve black and white food if you are a purist. Squid-ink spaghetti is served here with sour cream and caviar.

Fornasetti created no less than 500 versions of the same woman's face. These plates are precious but captivating and add humor to the mood of the table setting. There are many variations on the theme of black and white, each one different from the last. It can be interesting to keep a photographic record of each setting.

CONTEMPORARY
COLORS

A combination of rainbow colors and unusual shapes in this unique dinner service designed by Maryse Boxer ensures a richly patterned setting that can be varied according to occasion and season. Below, the juxtaposition of strong colors and sympathetic curves creates a dramatic, modern place setting.

The jewel-like quality of bright glassware and plastic-handled flatware brings a saturation of color to the overall effect of the table setting. The mixture of colored napkins, china, flowers, and glassware has an almost kaleidoscopic effect; patterns change with the progression of courses. Gerber daisies are ideal flowers as their shape and color are as emphatic as their surroundings.

LEFT *Lively combinations of color and shapes from Maryse Boxer's collection of rainbow-colored ceramics and tableware.*

CONTEMPORARY

CLASSICS

RIGHT *A detail of a coffee cup. Each course of the meal will effect a kaleidoscopic change in the color scheme.*

A place setting in a single yellow color tone with petal-shaped plates creates a strong block of color and looks effective next to the same setting in a different primary color. The combined textures of china, flatware, and napkin also contribute to the overall effect. The soft pleated napkin can be knotted, folded, or tucked inside a glass.

The right choice of food is both necessary and fun when using bright-colored ceramics or glass dishes. Salads, fruits — such as pears poached in red wine, below — sorbets, and most summer foods look delicious in these settings.

A combination of colored, hand-blown glass dishes and colored wineglasses are placed for the dessert course. Make use of the bright hues of summer fruits to build up color contrasts on the table.

A collection of primary colors or a mixture of primary and secondary colors — such as green or orange — will always create a dramatic table-scape. Increase the amount of contrasting color or a color you are short of with flowers and fruits of that color.

CONTEMPORARY

CLASSICS

This jumble of ceramics, flatware, and glassware in a myriad of shapes and colors demonstrates an effective blend of hues. Colors should be carefully selected so that the table setting does not jar. For example, the introduction of black, stone, or beige would not work here. Use paint cards to experiment with color before you begin a collection. Unless you plan to dazzle, a white tablecloth is a good background. This cloth is made of white organdy inset with tiny Indian-style mirrors, each bordered with different-colored silk.

RIGHT *A rainbow of color in flatware, glassware, and napkins suggests a kaleidoscope of combinations that will create a dramatic tabletop.*

TOP *A three-tier setting of heart-shaped plates set off by a sugar stick is perfect for a Valentine's Day supper.*

ABOVE *This place setting combines square and curved shapes in orange with red-handled cutlery. The knotted napkin nestles inside the bowl but drapes over each side and the flatware.*

CONTEMPORARY

CLASSICS

*A pleasing blend of
bright and soft colors of
glassware by Keith Rowe
is set upon a pale
turquoise table.*

*The individuality of hand-blown glass
makes a definitive statement when used on
the table or for display. Designs are often
remarkable and a slight irregularity of
shape makes a piece both charming and
distinctive. You can commission your own
glassware to a particular design or color. It
is not difficult to find unusual
contemporary glass at competitive prices. A
large individual serving or display plate or
a set of colored glasses will enhance any
dinner table. Again, effective color
combinations can almost achieve the
quality of a still life.*

*Use the juxtaposition of
colors to dramatic effect
– limes or lemons
against a bright-blue
glass dish and orange
Gerber daisies in a pale
turquoise vase.*

INFLUENCES FROM AFAR

We have always taken inspiration from other cultures, adapting their patterns, pottery, and precious metals to our own use. There are so many restaurants offering ethnic food and such a variety of imported ingredients that it is easy to experiment with exotic dishes. Enhancing the meal by providing an appropriate setting adds to the sense of occasion. So many fine tabletop items are imported from the Far East, Indonesia, the Mediterranean, Scandinavia, and many other regions that we are spoiled with choices. Collections from your favorite countries can be built up when you travel, which is great fun. Tablecloths made from colorful or exotic fabrics provide an effective background and offer more choice than traditional table linen. Lighting also creates atmosphere; a Mediterranean theme benefits from sunshine, while Moroccan and northern African settings look good with candlelit lanterns. Nordic wooden candelabra are charming, as are small Chinese table lanterns. Each table setting should reflect the influence of the chosen menu and the occasion.

CHINESE STYLE

Chinese food is very popular and many Westerners are now adept at eating with chopsticks. Chinese markets are a rich source of traditional tableware and ready-prepared foodstuffs. The poppy is a perfect flower for the table and injects color into the setting.

LEFT *Tableware from Chinatown is set upon a remnant of shantung with red chopsticks and vibrant poppies.*

RIGHT *A traditionally shaped yellow Chinese teapot, cup, and saucer set upon a teacloth appliquéd with bamboo and lanterns.*

There is a Chinatown in many large cities, where tableware, chopsticks, and cooking implements are readily available. The traditional colors, patterns, and symbols all have particular meanings. The theme of the design of this tableware is prosperity, longevity, and happiness.

Tea is usually served with the meal. A small drinking cup is provided as well as a bowl, spoon, plate, and chopsticks. Chopsticks are placed on a chopstick rest. The spoon has a flat bottom so it may be set down without spilling the contents. Individual bowls are used for rice.

RIGHT *These are the eating implements and tableware for one place setting. The teapot is shared.*

ABOVE *Chinese sweet cakes.*

LEFT *Chinese chopsticks (far left) are usually fashioned into blunt ends, while Japanese chopsticks (center) have pointed ends. On the right is a child's pair of lacquered Japanese chopsticks.*

Depending on the Chinese pattern you choose, the color scheme can be enhanced by the addition of flowers such as poppies, peonies, or jasmine. This tablecloth is fashioned from a length of shantung, and the napkin is chosen for its color and silken quality. However, napkins are not used in China nor in Chinese restaurants; hot towels are provided for face and hands.

MOROCCO BOUND

An abundance of decorated Moroccan pottery, Fes and Safi bowls, relish dishes, brass coffee-pots and tin teapots, colored mint tea glasses, tagine and couscous dishes, and brass plates heaped with typical Moroccan produce all work together to create a richly exotic setting for a delicious North African menu. In the background a wooden screen is positioned so as to dapple sunlight onto the table and seclude the diners. Traditionally food is taken with the fingers of the right hand. A perfume bottle is used to sprinkle rose water onto the hands.

RIGHT *Various glazed bowls and plates are set against the geometric blue-and-yellow-patterned food dishes and Safi pots.*

LEFT *A tagine dish, with an open funnel for steam, is accompanied by a traditional brass coffeepot.*

BELOW *The elements of one place setting are set on table linen embroidered with traditional geometric patterns. Elegant minaret-shaped mint teapots are in common use throughout Morocco. Teapots and glasses are not expensive and may be purchased easily in Moroccan "souks" or specialist shops.*

Bring together pottery, pots, brass plates, and wooden spoons you have collected that share common themes – good color combinations, shapes, metalwork, Islamic patterns – and create an exotic table setting.

LEFT *The blue-glass and decorated silver perfume shaker in the center of the table is used to shake rose water into the hands after eating. The toothpicks are made from dried flowers.*

RIGHT *Spices in little dishes, olives, dates, and oranges can be used to conjure up a sensual Moroccan setting.*

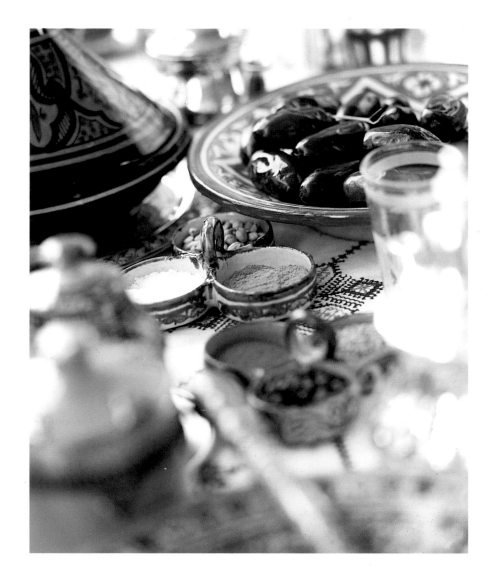

Blue geometric-patterned pottery is common in Morocco and blends well with English dark-blue-glazed pottery. These dishes may effectively be used as serving or dessert dishes.

MINT TEA

Everyone stops for mint tea. This refreshing and invigorating beverage is de rigueur and easy to make. It is an excellent after-dinner drink and cleanses the palate. Right, a tray of mint tea is set out at the famous El Minzah hotel in Tangier.

1 *Make mint tea as follows: Put two heaping teaspoonfuls of green tea into a small teapot.*

2 *Add a good handful of fresh mint, and as many spoonfuls of sugar as you require (it is usual to drink this tea extremely sweet, with as many as 12 spoonfuls of sugar added to the pot).*

3 *Pour on the boiling water.*

4 *Serve the tea in glasses. A sprig or two of fresh mint in the glass adds to the flavor and appearance.*

1

2

3

4

MEDITERRANEAN

The ideal setting is outside. A large jar of sunflowers reminiscent of Van Gogh establishes the scene, along with a mélange of rustic terra-cotta pottery, traditional honey-glazed bowls, heavy ceramic pottery with a blue glaze and floral design, generously sized glasses, a gaily colored tablecloth, a few breadsticks, a jug or two of wine, cheese, salad, and good weather. Marigolds or any country flowers in season add to the overall color scheme. Line baskets with checked or brightly colored plain napkins and fill with rolls, tomatoes, or whole salad fruits. Then imagine yourself in the warm Mediterranean sun.

LEFT A single place setting mixes terracotta from Portugal, a modern Quimper plate, and a traditional honey-glazed Provençal bowl. The tableware is set upon a length of turquoise Designers Guild fabric with large naive floral motifs.

Select rustic tableware, café-style flatware, and colored glasses, and serve simple fare such as onion quiche and tomato and olive salad.

RIGHT Place the knife and fork to the right of the place setting in an informal style. This is useful if space is tight.

RIGHT *Various types of Mediterranean pottery are used in one place setting.*

BELOW *Goat cheese garnished with pink peppercorns makes an effective foil for a blue-glazed plate.*

The common theme among these settings is the rustic feel of the ceramics, which, although quite at odds in color and pattern, are similar in texture and weight.

ALFRESCO

*E*ating outside is fun, whether it's a simple family
barbecue on the patio, a summer lunch party, a
wedding feast, or a picnic at an outdoor event. It can be
formal or informal according to the occasion, but it is
inevitably jolly and never fails to generate high spirits, even
in the least likely guest. Everyone may bring a particular item
of food and tableware, which usually ensures an element of
surprise when the cloth is spread. Passionate picnickers have
special hampers replete with china and flatware, ready-
packed for impromptu opportunities on sunny days. Such a
set can be quickly put together with simple colored plates, an
assortment of glasses, cheerful gingham linen, and tin or
enamel mugs. A fold-up table and chairs are useful, or take
your cue from Manet and sit on the grass.

PICNIC

TIME

A colorful gingham cloth catches the breeze at the beach. A galvanized bucket tied with a polka-dotted red hankie and weighted with pebbles serves as a wine cooler. Rough pieces of driftwood or sea-worn breakwaters make useful shelves for food baskets, and small mussel or cockle shells can be filled with seasonings such as salt. A tin milk pitcher, filled with red anemones, is anchored to the table with pebbles. The only problem remaining is to finish the meal before the tide comes in.

LEFT *A simple color scheme of red, white, and blue. A small stone keeps the gingham napkin on its plate.*

RIGHT *What better setting could there be for a picnic complete with champagne, flowers, and an improvised wine cooler.*

The key to a successful setting of this kind is to keep the color scheme simple and bright. Nothing should be too precious, as breakages are inevitable. The floor-length tablecoth is sewn from two lengths of gingham and has matching napkins. It is useful to have insect covers for food, especially in hot climates. Flowers may seem too much trouble to bring, but they provide a wonderful splash of color and create a sense of occasion.

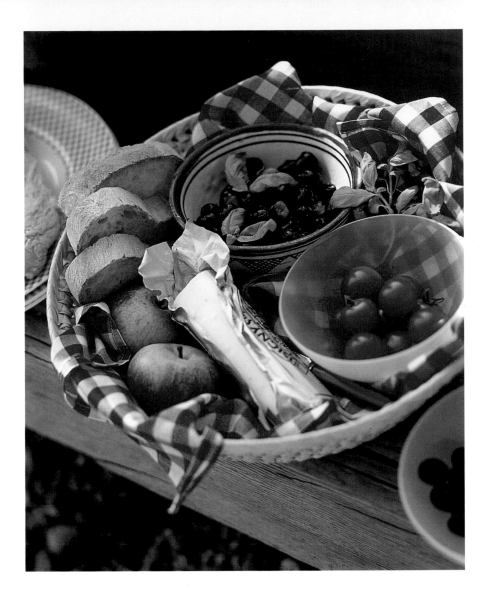

ABOVE *A breakwater beam serves as a shelf for a basket of food. Line baskets with napkins to keep food clean and to continue the festive theme.*

LEFT *A white linen napkin embroidered with red checks especially for the picnic hamper.*

LEFT *A detail of a single place setting in a red, white, and blue color scheme.*

LEFT *Picnic food is usually eaten cold, and part of the joy is not to stand on ceremony but to eat certain things with your fingers. The pitcher is anchored by rocks in case the wind blows.*

RIGHT *This simple but effective setting mixes checks and stripes in red, white, and blue.*

Simple, colorful table linen and tableware work well on a picnic table or spread upon the ground. Combine checks, stripes, polka-dots, and solid colors in your chosen color scheme. Flowers, napkins, and bread baskets are the extra touches that make the event special.

Picnics are informal gatherings – you can either sit around a picnic table or spread a blanket or tablecloth on the ground. Finger foods are the order of the day, and a ripe Brie and tomatoes complement the color scheme.

SORBET
COLORS

Eating outside is one of the joys that summer brings. Make the most of late sunsets, scented gardens, sea views, and the holiday atmosphere. Leisurely weekend lunches and summer suppers may be set up on a deck, terrace, patio, roof garden, balcony, on the lawn, or just by an open window. This atmosphere can be created or augmented by the evocative summer colors of a special dinner service. Here, pale frosted sorbet colors set the scene.

ABOVE *A tower of frosted resin sorbet dishes and matching spoon.*

RIGHT *A waterlily floats in each bowl, bringing symbols of summer to the table.*

Variations of frosted

pastel hues create a

delicate summer

table setting.

One place setting in various pastel tones set with the central vase of waterlilies.

The delicate colors of this table setting create soft combinations that complement and reflect the pale blue ocean beyond. Build upon this delicacy with pale-colored or white flowers and a white or organza cloth and napkins. Flatware with glass or colored handles would work well. Each place setting here has its own condiment set, and this helps to cover the table with patterns of color.

Contrast the colors of the sorbet with the colors of the dishes.

RIGHT *The elements used in one table setting are, clockwise from the top: bowl, bread-and-butter plate and butter knife, water and wine glass, sorbet dish and spoon, napkin and ring, and dinner plate with spoon and fork.*

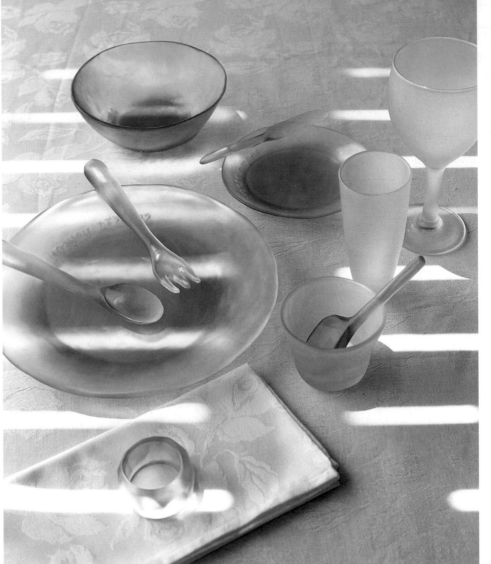

BELOW *The summer menu should suit the setting. Here a ripe peach makes a pleasing contrast set against frosted blue.*

Glass and similar materials (such as the frosted resin from Dinosaur Designs featured here) create a light, delicate setting. If the sun shines through them, colored shadow patterns appear on the table, which adds to the general effect. Waterlilies are particularly attractive floating in each bowl, but other large-headed flowers in bright colors would serve the same purpose.

SPECIAL OCCASIONS

Throughout life there are ritual celebrations to mark special occasions – christenings, birthdays, engagements, weddings, and anniversaries. In all societies there are festivals and feasts associated with the progress of the seasons and the religious calendar – New Year's, Valentine's Day, Easter, Thanksgiving, and Christmas. Each occasion requires attention to detail and planning of the menu, seating arrangements, and table setting. Flowers are always an excellent addition and add wonderful splashes of color to the plainest dinner service. These occasions present an ideal opportunity to polish silver, delve deep into china cupboards, light candles, bring on the champagne, fill the house with flowers, and prepare to make merry.

BEGGARS' BANQUET

A celebratory banquet at home is an appealing idea but seldom happens because of the expense. Here is an idea for a "banquet on a shoestring" that requires minimal outlay but lots of energy, enthusiasm, and innovative ideas. White sheets are used as tablecloths and enamel pitchers and mugs as vases with basic white china and stainless steel flatware for the setting. Trestle tables and "opera" chairs can be rented from a catering company.

RIGHT *Utilitarian trestle table and gold-backed chairs are rented for a cheerful "banquet" at home.*

A simple, functional
banquet setting can
be easily and
economically put
together with basic
tableware, flatware,
and drinking glasses
set off by generous
bunches of eye-
catching blue iris.

It is easier to get a lot of guests seated if a place card is put at each setting. Here they are placed inside the wineglasses as the atmosphere is informal. Place settings may be cramped, and carefully crossing flatware within the bowl creates some extra room. No bread plates are necessary; bread may be broken and left on

the table. Napkins are folded and placed under each bowl. If the trestle tables are narrow, it may help to present food buffet-style on a sideboard to be carried back to their places by the diners. Large pitchers of flowers can be removed, leaving the shorter arrangements in mugs for color.

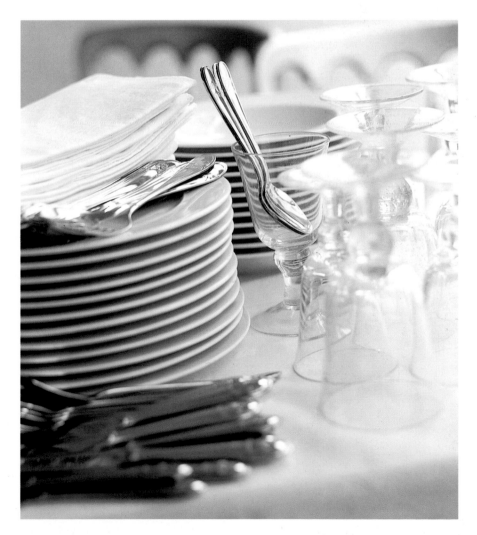

ABOVE *An effective crossed flatware arrangement for a cramped table setting.*

RIGHT *Simplicity of form, texture, and color is the key to this setting.*

The necessary accessories
are sheets to use as
tablecloths, enamel pitchers
(obtainable from hardware
stores), salt and pepper for
two or three guests to share,
and colorful flowers.

ABOVE *Wineglasses can
be used for desserts such as
sorbets or fruit compotes.*

RIGHT *One place setting
in detail.*

Large, informal dinner parties need to run smoothly, and it is therefore best to serve food that does not have to be prepared at the last minute, requires minimal attention once it is cooked, and looks appetitizing on a white plate. Puréed vegetable soups or mixed salads with varied ingredients – radicchio, green bell peppers, baby yellow tomatoes, sliced red onions, black olives – are ideal to start. This Warm Chicken Salad is also a perfect choice; serve it with a crisp white wine. Keep desserts simple and brightly colored to end on a cheery note – sorbets and ice creams are always crowd pleasers. Bright orange mango sorbet looks wonderful with fresh raspberries and sprigs of fresh mint leaves.

GRAND BUFFET LUNCH

Historically, a buffet meal was always laid out on a sideboard (the French word for this piece of furniture is still buffet*). Guests help themselves from the food offered and carry it to the table or sit down with plates on their laps. If you plan a buffet for many guests, a spectacular central display in a hall or large room creates a gathering place and a talking point which helps put people at their ease. Smaller displays echoing the main theme may be set up off to the side and chairs placed in small clusters around tables or in groups around the room to encourage mingling.*

A large still-life display is set on a trestle table with a Flemish tapestry as a backdrop for a grand buffet.

This display is unashamedly inspired by the great Dutch still-life painters Van Os and Van Huysum, and others such as Velázquez. Art books specializing in the genre, catalogs of exhibitions, and postcards are rich sources of ideas. Long before rooms were set aside especially for dining, meals were set upon trestles and boards covered with cloths, heavy draperies, leather, or carpets, as can be seen in the paintings. Here those textures are emulated with a bright blue damask and two Victorian chenille table covers. Three boxes are placed underneath the covers to create different heights for display (see picture on page 93).

The juxtaposition of fruits and other textures work well in this setting. For maximum effect, combine unlikely and evocative elements and make visual puns such as the mandarin oranges in the blue and white china bowl.

LEFT *Plates are piled up and knives and forks are wrapped in individual napkins folded tuxedo-style; instructions are on page 138.*

ABOVE *Artichokes, cabbage, and quails' eggs on a pewter plate are evocative of a still-life painting.*

The focal point of this still life is the spectacular display of flowers, fruit, and vegetables. The receptacle is a plastic pot placed inside a large terracotta plant pot. Three blocks of florist's foam are placed inside with water.

1

2

3

FLORAL DISPLAY:
1 *Find a postcard of a still life you wish to copy and make notes about its structure. Place the stems of foliage, berries, and trailing ivy into the florist's foam first, following your skeleton structure.*

2 *Place the flowers, vegetables, and fruit in position. Artichoke stems can be wedged straight in, while fruits such as pomegranates or pineapples need to be pierced with florist's wire which is then stuck into the foam.*

3 *Fill out the naturally occurring holes with the remaining flowers, referring constantly to your inspirational painting.*

Flower stems are pierced into the foam and unwieldy fruits such as pineapples are threaded with thick florist's wire and held in position in the same way. In many paintings butterflies, small birds, or a snail can be seen. Models of such creatures could be added to the display.

*This detail of the
arrangement shows,
among other things,
parrot tulips, an
artichoke, a pineapple,
berries, lilies, red
ranunculus, and
delphiniums.*

BYZANTIUM

This lavishly adorned tableware – created by Peter Crisp – features slumped glass bowls and plates, silk-screened with various ornamental patterns in 22-carat gold, indigo, and green. These embellished plates and bowls are objects of art in themselves. The combination of gold and glass is startling and can be enhanced by candlelight to evoke romantic mood. The silverware, known as the Crisp design, was created and crafted by Lyndsey Davey especially to complement the tableware. Gardenias bring a heavy fragrance to the table.

LEFT *A polished
refectory table set with
this unique glassware
and silverware.
Individual place mats
allow the grain and
beauty of the wood to
enhance the opulence of
this setting and reflect
the glow of candlelight.
Gardenias bring their
own unique fragrance.*

ABOVE *Gold upon gold
– in glass or as a border
on china – makes a rich
table setting.*

ABOVE *Combine old and new with this Victorian silver and blue-glass salt and pepper set.*

ABOVE RIGHT *A single place setting for a three-course meal, including soup. The soup spoons are fashioned in the French style, with an oval bowl and pointed tip.*

Accessories for a dinner party based upon the grand theme of gold, glass, silver, and creamy-whites. Clockwise from the left are decanters and glass candle holders sparkling by candlelight, a candelabra and parchment-colored beeswax candles, creamy, scented gardenias and silver napkin rings.

As always, the menu should be planned with the setting in mind. The pale green of the cold asparagus soup goes well with the gold patterns on the dishes. Rich dark chocolate cake and a generous helping of cream suits gold as does the liquid gold of a good dessert wine.

Gold and silver go together. Left, an effective setting for a special occasion can be achieved with gold-rimmed china plates and silver flatware and accessories. The gardenia adds a finishing touch. Right, the requirements for one place setting. Note the large soup spoon at the bottom of the picture.

LEFT *Turn breakfast into a special occasion with an ornate eggcup and matching spoon set with mock pearls.*

RIGHT *This silver napkin ring features the guest's name.*

CHRISTMAS DAY

Christmas offers an excellent opportunity to create a festive table setting. It is the one occasion for which many families reserve special tablecloths, centerpieces, and napkins. The table is usually laden with candles, small gifts, and decorative objects. Traditional color schemes are green, red, and white. Red is always warm and welcoming. However, this table setting is inspired by the colors of Christmas roses and mistletoe. Warmth emanates from firelight and candles. A collection of white plates is a must for every china cupboard, as it can be combined with any color. Silk damask is used as a tablecloth and the chargers are tin cooking plates.

LEFT *Posies of
Christmas roses,
mistletoe, ivy, and
rosemary arranged in
green glass dessert dishes
create a light, refreshing
centerpiece at each place
setting.*

BELOW *Frosty themes
of green, silver, and
white for a Christmas
setting.*

*Typical accessories for a
Christmas setting
include tree ornaments,
miniature English
Christmas crackers, and
candles in appropriate
colors. Build up the
collection of colors,
adding gold for glitter,
and varying the shades
of green.*

The elements of one table setting. The dessert dish holds the Christmas posy.

This Christmas setting does not require a large investment; the elements may be collected together at relatively little expense. Green recycled glassware, pictured here, is now widely available, and the tin dishes used as chargers are easily found in hardware stores. These dishes can be effectively "pewterized" by baking them in a hot oven for half an hour. White or green napkins are equally effective, or a symbol of Christmas, such as a sprig of mistletoe, could be embroidered onto one corner. Decorate napkins with Christmas greens and berries.

1 *For napkin decoration you will need a pair of wire cutters, florist's wire, a piece of ivy, and a sprig of mistletoe.*

2 *Twist florist's wire around the napkin and weave ivy over and under it. Secure the ends under the wire at the back.*

3 *Tuck mistletoe or berries under the wire to secure. Warning: ivy and mistletoe are poisonous and should not used for small children's napkins.*

You will need a vase, clippers, and sprigs of choisya, ivy, mistletoe, freesia, Christmas roses, and rosemary.

Fill the dish with water. Place four pieces of choisya around the rim, then put four pieces of ivy in between.

Place bunches of rosemary between the choisya and ivy. Add two sprigs of mistletoe at four equal points.

Add four white Christmas roses and four white freesia, spacing them equally. Jasmine or other greenery with feathery leaves can be used to fill out the posy.

A posy bowl at each

place setting

establishes an

intimate and

welcoming

atmosphere and

creates the

impression of

attention to detail.

CANDLELIT SUPPER FOR TWO

This supper is intended for a romantic occasion – an anniversary, Valentine's Day, or a special celebration. The color scheme is gold and silver, with cream and white roses, which are scattered on shelves and tucked into each napkin. If you prefer traditional red roses, another color of tablecloth such as dusky pink would be suitable. The room is lit with slow-burning candles.

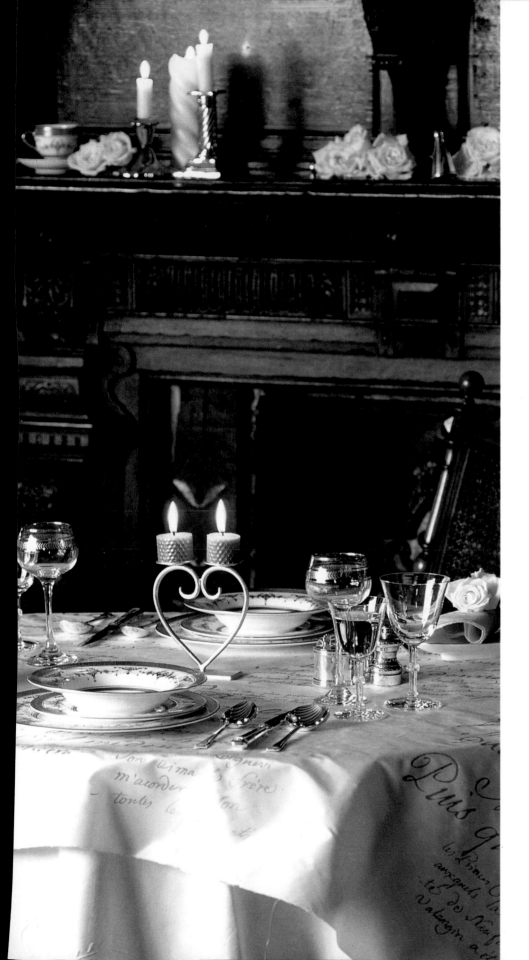

LEFT *The setting for a candlelit supper for two using a color scheme of gold, silver, cream, and white.*

ABOVE *A romantic heart-shaped candle holder – the perfect symbol of Valentine's Day.*

ABOVE *A collection of white, parchment, and barley-twist candles and holders. Don't forget to include a candle snuffer.*

RIGHT *A single place setting in Minton's Riverton service. A single creamy rose tucked inside the silver napkin ring adds to the decorative effect. A crescent-shape salad plate is placed to the left of the setting.*

A romantic supper for two at home has to be planned well and this may be difficult if the occasion is to be a surprise. As there will only be two of you, the less last-minute cooking the better. A cold hors d'œuvre such as oysters and a cold dessert are recommended, plus a simple main course such as baked salmon fillet.

BELOW *A novel and very personal idea for dessert would be a miniature frosted chocolate sponge cake decorated with white roses.*

RIGHT *Silver and gold accessories are used and set upon a "tablecloth" of handmade silk-screened fabric by Carolyn Quartermaine. Also suitable would be white damask or white linen, embroidered with gold thread.*

FLORIBUNDA

*F*lowers are not only wonderful used fresh as table decorations, but are frequently the inspiration behind the design of dinner and tea services. Tablecloths, napkins, and tea cozies are often woven or embroidered with floral motifs; even flatware handles are sometimes embossed with flowers. Flowers are a simple and appealing theme to use as the basis of a table setting, which can be subtle and monotonal or extravagant and wildly colorful. Here rose heads are woven into garden chairs, and petals are cast, like confetti, over the terrace. A pretty coffee set on a white lace-bordered tablecloth helps to set a captivating afternoon scene.

TEA AND ROSES

This color scheme is based on soft tones. The juxtaposition of Regency stripes, pink roses in two shades, green frosted glass, and a silver teapot and cake stand, all set upon a delicate embroidered organza tablecloth (over plain pink fabric which shows through), creates a soft, fresh setting.

FLORIBUNDA

FAR LEFT *Tea with scones, clotted cream, and strawberry jam.*

LEFT *In the pink for afternoon tea. Even the cakes complement the color scheme.*

Cut rose stems and plunge them immediately into water. If you wish them to open quickly, plunge them into warm water, with an aspirin to make them last longer. Buy or pick roses a few days beforehand if you want them to open and create a generous, almost full-blown, display.

1

2

1 *Sew tiny ribbon rosebuds onto a white tablecloth for a rosy effect. These little silk or satin decorations, which are frequently used in dressmaking, are available in many delicate colors. They create a busy background against which plain white plates can look striking.*

2 *Place a white cloth on the table you intend to decorate. Work out where each place setting will be, then sew the buds around the edges of the cloth and in the center.*

A cake stand is de rigueur at afternoon tea and enhances the display by offsetting and balancing the height of the flowers. Sandwich fillings of cucumber and smoked salmon match the color scheme.

FLORIBUNDA

Only a few pieces of this tea service remain, but a rosy patchwork effect is created by combining these with a contemporary silver teapot and creamer and fresh roses. Echo the rose theme in the posy, and make a rosebud-chain napkin ring. The pastry forks embossed with roses were a very lucky find.

Pieces of a pretty Victorian tea service with contemporary silver teapot and creamer.

Start a collection of floral-decorated plates with a color bias – such as a pink or pale blue background – and soon you will have a tea or dinner service. As flowers are such a popular theme, new or revived designs are frequently launched.

A selection of Limoges plates with floral patterns.

BREAKFAST
IN BED

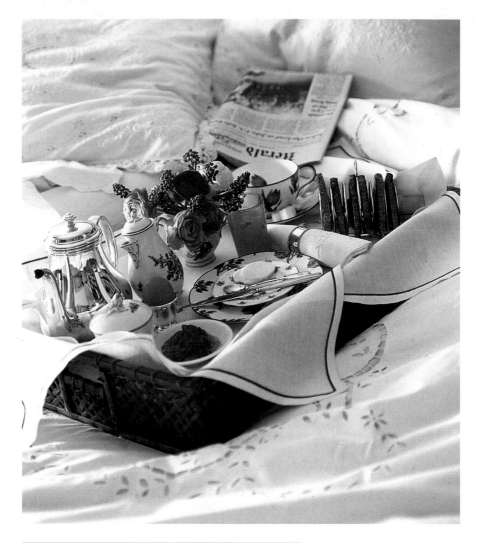

Breakfast is usually such a hurried meal, if eaten at all, that most people consider it a real luxury to be brought breakfast in bed on the weekend. You will need a large, sturdy tray or a purpose-built tray on a folding stand. A flower theme and a colorful posy provide a cheerful morning greeting. Keep toast or rolls warm under cloths and a cozy on the teapot. Here the menu consists of grapefruit juice, a soft-boiled egg, toast, butter, home-made marmalade, and a pot of English Breakfast tea.

ABOVE *A large breakfast tray set with a colorful mixture of plates, pots, and cups featuring floral patterns.*

RIGHT *Pink ranunculus and grape hyacinths echo the flower arrangement depicted on the adjacent Dresden pitcher.*

DAYS OF WINE AND ROSES

Deep red roses set the tone for this elegant and substantial setting. The rose-patterned china echoes rose-embossed silverware, and the motif is repeated on the etched wineglasses and embroidered organza napkins. Everywhere the eye falls upon a rosy image. Every piece on the table is chosen for quality and elegance. Red and white rose petals scattered around create a festive atmosphere. Napkins are folded into a variation of the bishop's miter (see page 138 for instructions) and rosé wine is served.

RIGHT *Another variation on the theme of roses. Folded organza napkins lend an air of formality and define each place setting.*

FLORIBUNDA

OVERLEAF *The full table setting for a rose-themed formal dinner party.*

ABOVE *"Rose" silverware embossed with trailing roses, which also appear in delicate relief on the front and back of the spoon.*

APPENDIX

This Appendix includes a guide to international table settings and their variations, types of drinking glasses, and a visual glossary of the more common flatware pieces. It also offers ideas for napkin folding and place cards. The Appendix is intended not as the definitive word on etiquette but merely as a guide.

1

ENGLISH FORMAL

The accepted procedure for laying a table is knives on the right and forks on the left. Soup spoons are placed on the outside right of knives and dessert spoons on the inside right. Sometimes the dessert spoon and fork are laid horizontally above the plate (see page 130). If in doubt, work from the outside inward, according to the order of courses. Sometimes a smaller, additional knife is placed on the bread plate or on the outside right of the setting. The bread plate is to the left of the forks.

1. BREAD-AND-BUTTER PLATE
   (SIDE PLATE)
2. NAPKIN IN A SIMPLE FOLD
3. TABLE OR DINNER FORK
4. DESSERT FORK
5. PLACE CARD
6. DINNER PLATE
7. FROM LEFT TO RIGHT, WATER GLASS,
   RED-WINE GLASS, AND WHITE-WINE GLASS
8. DESSERT SPOON
9. TABLE OR DINNER KNIFE
10. SOUP SPOON

2

SETTING FOR A CROWDED TABLE

If space around the dinner table is cramped, the bread-and-butter plate may be dispensed with and the napkin placed upon the dinner plate. The dessert spoon and fork are laid horizontally above the setting with the fork tines pointing toward the knife (right) and the spoon bowl toward the fork (left). If other eating implements are necessary, they can accompany their courses.

1. TABLE FORK	4. DESSERT FORK	7. WHITE-WINE GLASS
2. DINNER PLATE	5. DESSERT SPOON	8. TABLE KNIFE
3. NAPKIN	6. RED-WINE GLASS	9. SOUP SPOON

3

AMERICAN FORMAL

In an American setting the bread plate is set above the forks. If a butter knife is provided, it may be laid to the side of or above the bread plate. Both knife and fork are used to cut food, but the fork may be transferred to the right hand for eating.

1. NAPKIN
2. FIRST-COURSE FISH FORK
3. DINNER FORK
4. DESSERT FORK
5. BREAD-AND-BUTTER PLATE
6. DINNER PLATE
7. WATER GLASS
8. RED-WINE GLASS
9. WHITE-WINE GLASS
10. DESSERT SPOON
11. DINNER KNIFE
12. FISH KNIFE

4

FRENCH
FORMAL

In a traditional setting, forks and spoons lie face down (originally to show the family crest). Sometimes knives are rested upon a porte-couteau (knife rest). Soup spoons are oval with a pointed end, except for consommé. Butter is never served with bread, so butter knives are not required. However, both a knife and fork are used to eat cheese, which is served after the main course (with the same red wine as the main course) and before dessert.

1. DINNER FORK
2. DESSERT FORK
3. DINNER PLATE
4. NAPKIN
5. SALT AND PEPPER SET
6. WATER GLASS

7. RED-WINE GLASS
8. WHITE-WINE GLASS
9. DESSERT SPOON
10. DINNER KNIFE
11. CONSOMMÉ SPOON
12. PORTE-COUTEAU

5

ITALIAN FORMAL

A formal Italian table setting depends upon the order in which the food is to be served, and whether there is pasta, fish, or soup first. If in doubt, work from the outside in, or wait for your host to select his or her implements before you begin. In this setting the fork on the far right is for risotto (first course), which is to be followed by fish and then meat.

1. FISH FORK
2. DINNER FORK (MAIN COURSE)
3. SALT AND PEPPER SET
4. DINNER PLATE
5. NAPKIN
6. RED-WINE GLASS
7. WHITE-WINE GLASS
8. DINNER KNIFE
9. FISH KNIFE
10. PASTA OR RISOTTO FORK

6

CHINESE FORMAL

The popularity of Chinese food has encouraged Westerners to use chopsticks. However, it is considerate to offer a spoon and fork as well to guests who may not have mastered the art. Rice is served into bowls by the host and people serve themselves the rest of the food from central bowls, but not using their chopsticks. It is not polite to "fish around" in the serving dish or attempt to cut food. If a morsel of food is too large it should be separated from other items and eaten on its

own. The flat-bottomed spoon is used for soup or more slippery food.

1. TEACUP
2. BOWL AND SAUCER
3. TEAPOT
4. DINNER PLATE
5. SOUP SPOON
6. CHOPSTICKS
7. CHOPSTICK REST
8. LOW BAMBOO TABLE

GLASSES

7

FOR EVERY OCCASION

A good supply of red- and white-wine glasses together with tall and short glasses for mineral waters, soft drinks, and spirits is usually sufficient for a dinner party. Goblets or tumblers (whichever look more attractive with the setting) are suitable for mineral water. Glasses are grouped on the right of the setting above the blade of the longest knife. The usual procedure is to place the first-course glass nearest the diner. For example, the small white-wine glass that accompanies

the first course (which may be fish) is placed on the outside right. If other glasses are required, they can accompany the course for which they are intended, especially if space is short.

1   2   3   4   5   6   7   8   9

1. GOBLET
2. CHAMPAGNE FLUTE
3. LARGE WINE (RED)
4. WINE (WHITE)
5. SHERRY
6. LIQUEUR
7. HIGHBALL GLASS
8. OLD-FASHIONED GLASS
9. BRANDY

FLATWARE

FOR EVERY PURPOSE

The Victorians invented an eating implement for every possible occasion. Its particular function was often to prevent the fingers from touching food. The Victorians are responsible for fish knives and forks, for example, which have been in continuous use for more than 100 years (but were considered vulgar in certain circles). If you enjoy collecting silver, the chances are most of the decorative utensils you find will be Victorian. There are a variety of soup spoons for different soups, as well as jam, tea, coffee, trifle, caviar,

1   2   3   4   5   6   7

1   2   3   4   5   6   7   8   9   10

and egg spoons. There are snail and pastry forks, and forks for every seafood imaginable. Originally, one knife (which the diner carried on his person) was used with bread as a "pusher". Individual forks began to be used in the 17th century. Early forks had two tines. "Silver" was used to describe eating utensils, for obvious reasons, but "flatware" is now the accepted term in the United States, "cutlery" in Britain.

KNIVES

1. TABLE OR DINNER KNIFE
2. STEAK KNIFE (WITH SERRATED EDGE)
3. CAVIAR KNIFE (WITH HORN BLADE)
4. TEA KNIFE
5. DESSERT KNIFE
6. FISH KNIFE
7. BUTTER KNIFE

FORKS

1. TABLE OR DINNER FORK
2. EARLY FORK WITH THREE TINES
3. STEAK FORK
4. FISH FORK
5. DESSERT FORK
6. FRUIT FORK
7. TEA FORK
8. PASTRY FORK
9. SNAIL FORK
10. OYSTER FORK

SPOONS

1. SERVING SPOON
2. DESSERT SPOON
3. ENGLISH SOUP SPOON
4. TRIFLE SPOON
5. ICE-CREAM SPOON
6. FRUIT SPOON
7. GRAPEFRUIT SPOON
8. TEASPOON
9. COFFEE SPOON
10. DEMITASSE COFFEE SPOON

TABLE NAPKINS

9

THE ART OF FOLDING

Fashions in the folding of napkins come and go. In the 17th century it was considered an art, and at Versailles napkins were folded into many shapes, including boats, chickens with eggs, and peacocks. It was a breach of etiquette to demolish these, so fresh napkins were supplied for use during the meal. Emily Post in the 1920s declared "fancy foldings are not in good taste," but today folded napkins, appropriate to the occasion are decorative.

TUXEDO FOLD	BISHOP'S MITER	JAPANESE FOLD	PEACOCK'S TAIL

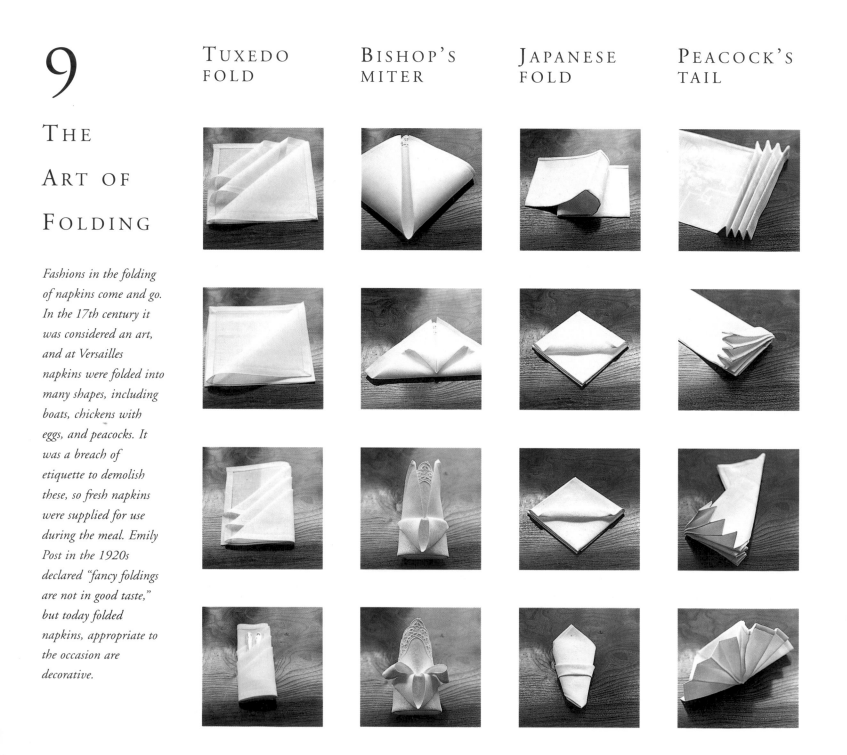

PLACE CARDS

10

THE ART OF LABELING

If there are more than a few guests it simplifies seating arrangements to put place card at each setting. For a formal dinner, small fancy place card holders, such as the miniature silver pears above left, can be found at many good tableware stores. Another novel idea is to tie a place card to the stem of a piece of real or carved fruit. This works well at wedding receptions, with golden fruit and heart-shaped place cards. Or lay a flower tied with a velvet ribbon and the place card on a dinner plate.

DIRECTORY OF SOURCES

BLUE AND WHITE

FRENCH BISTRO, pages 10 -15
Selection of plates and glasses from Jerry's Home Store.
Silver condiment set from Thomas Goode.
Milk jug from Bridgewater Pottery, China & Glass

ASIATIC PHEASANT, pages 16-21
'Asiatic pheasant' crockery collected at antique fairs
and markets.
'New' Asiatic Pheasant from Burgess & Leigh.

HARLEQUIN BLUE, pages 22-27
Table linen from The White House
Cake stand from Royal Copenhagen at Georg Jensen
Blue and white china from Spode and private collections
Blue hock, wine and water glasses and selected
silverware from Thomas Goode

CONTEMPORARY CLASSICS

CLASSIC GOLD, pages 30-35
Selected table linen, cruet, decanters,
dinner service from Thomas Goode.
Cutlery by Christofle.
Selected glassware from Lalique.

BLACK AND WHITE, pages 36 - 41
Cloth on tables, The Renaissance Collection,
and 'Lionman' plate from Timney Fowler.
Candelabra, vases and 'Moser' wine glasses from
Thomas Goode.
Fornasetti china and selected cutlery from
Rosenthal studio-haus.
Chopsticks from Maryse Boxer at Chez Joseph.

CONTEMPORARY COLORS, pages 42-49
Rainbow coloured tableware - plates, cutlery and glasses
in coral, turquoise, purple and yellow all by Maryse
Boxer at Chez Joseph.
Hand-blown coloured glassware by Keith Rowe.

INFLUENCES FROM AFAR

CHINESE STYLE, pages 52 -55
Chinese bowls, teapot and chopsticks from
Chinatown, London WC2

MOROCCO BOUND, pages 56 - 63
Most items from The Kasbah.
Mint tea service provided by and photographed at
El Minzah Hotel, Tangier.

MEDITTERANEAN, pages 64 - 69
Tablecloth fabric, 'Kasuti', napkins, gingham basket
and selected plates from Designers Guild.
Selected terracotta, yellow, blue plates and cutlery
from Divertimenti.
Selected rustic bowls, terracotta, 'Quimper' plates and
blue goblets from Elizabeth David.

ALFRESCO

PICNIC TIME, pages 72 - 77
Selected hampers, blue glasses and table plates from
Jerry's Home Store.

SORBET COLORS, pages 78 - 82
Frosted pastel resin (hand-moulded) dinner service from
Dinosaur Designs.

SPECIAL OCCASIONS

BEGGARS' BANQUET, pages 86 -91
Plates, cutlery and glasses from IKEA

GRAND BUFFET LUNCH, pages 92 -97
Flemish tapestry from Joanna Booth.
Silver dishes, claret jug, horn-handled knives and forks
from Mappin & Webb.
Chenille cloths from Gallery of Antique Costume &
Textiles.

BYZANTIUM, pages 98 - 103
Slumped glass and gold dishes by Peter Crisp from
The Crisp Galleries
"The Crisp Design" Hand crafted silver cutlery by
Lindsay Davy.
China, drinking glasses and selected cutlery from
Country Road Homeware
Eggcup and spoons set with pearls from
Victoria Spring Designs.

CHRISTMAS DAY, pages 104 - 109
Bone china white dinner service 'White Traditional'
from Wedgwood.

CANDLELIT SUPPER FOR TWO, pages 110 - 113
Bone china 'Riverton' dinner service by Minton.
'Beaugency' glassware by Lalique.
Cutlery by United Cutlers
Heart-shaped candle holder from
Maryse Boxer at Chez Joseph.
Silk-screen printed fabric by
Carolyn Quartermaine at Chez Joseph.

FLORIBUNDA

pages 114-115
Victorian fretwork garden chairs from Appley Hoare.

TEA AND ROSES, pages 116 - 121
Silver teapot c. 1818, jar and spoon from Garrard.
'Carousel' tea service, cake stand,
'Marie Antoinette' and 'Laure Selignac'
Limoges plates from Thomas Goode.
Tablecloth and table napkins from The White House.

BREAKFAST IN BED pages 122-123
Embroidered napkins used as tray cloth and silver
napkin ring from Thomas Goode.
Raynaud 'Jardin de Villandry' tea plate, breakfast cup
and saucer and Christofle 'Bagatelle' silver teapot
from Asprey.
Dresden 'Mocha' set from Garrard.

DAYS OF WINE AND ROSES, pages 124 - 127
Victorian iron children's table and chairs
from Appley Hoare Antiques
Napkins and tablecloth from Lunn Antiques
Rose patterned china by Richard Ginori from ICTC.
'Rose' silver embossed cutlery and Murano wine glasses
'Doves and flowers' from Asprey.

INTERNATIONAL TABLE SETTINGS, GLASSES
AND CUTLERY Pages 130 - 137
Dinner plates from Thomas Goode.
Selected cutlery from Mappin & Webb
Glassware 'Monterrey' from Stuart Crystal.

PLACE CARDS page 139
Small silver pear name-card holder from Asprey.
Miniature iced cake from Patisserie Valerie.
All white china (apart from pages 86-91) by Wedgwood.

THE WHITE HOUSE
51 -52 New Bond Street
London W1Y OBY
Telephone: 0171 629 3521

SPODE
Church Street
Stoke-on-Trent, ST4 1BX
Telephone: 01782 744011

ROYAL COPENHAGEN
AT GEORG JENSEN
15 New Bond Street
London W1
Telephone: 0171 499 6541

THOMAS GOODE &
CO. (LONDON) LTD.
19 South Audley Street
London W1Y 6BN
Telephone: 0171 499 2823

JERRY'S HOME STORE
163-167 Fulham Road
London SW3 6SN
Telephone: 0171 581 0909

BRIDGEWATER
POTTERY CHINA
& GLASS
739 Fulham Road
London SW6 5UL
Telephone: 0171 371 9033

ASIATIC PHEASANT
(current production) Customer
enquiries
BURGESS & LEIGH
Middleport Pottery
Port Street, Burslem
Stoke-on-Trent
ST6 3PE
Telephone: 01782 577 866

CHRISTOFLE
SILVERWARE
10 Hanover Street
London W1R 9HF
Telephone: 0171 491 4004

TIMNEY FOWLER
388 Kings Road
London SW3 5UZ
Telephone: 0171 352 2263

ROSENTHAL
(STUDIO-HAUS)
Goldsmith House
137 Regent Street
London W1R 8ND
Telephone: 0171 734 0727

MARYSE BOXER AT
CHEZ JOSEPH
26 Sloane Street
London SW1 7LQ
0171 245 9493
(also at Barney's New York,
Conran, Paris and
The Bay Tree, Sydney)

KEITH ROWE
Hand blown glass
Unit 7
134 Station Street
Blackheath
NSW 2785
PO BOX 219
BLACK HEATH NSW 2785
Telephone: 047 9877 220

VICTORIA SPRING
DESIGNS
Handmade jewellery and
tableware
33 William Street
Paddington
Sydney
NSW 2021
Telephone: 61 2 9331 7862

APPLEY HOARE
ANTIQUES
55 Queen Street
Woollahra
Sydney
NSW 2025
Telephone: 61 2 9362 3045

CHINATOWN
LISLE AND GERRARD
STREET, NEWPORT
COURT AREAS
Soho London WC2

THE KASBAH
8 Southampton Street
London WC2
Telephone: 0171 240 3538

ELIZABETH DAVID
North Row, The Piazza
Covent Garden, London WC2
Telephone: 0171 938 9167

DIVERTIMENTI
139 Fulham Road
London SW3 6SD
Telephone: 0171 581 8065

DESIGNERS GUILD
267 -272 & 277 Kings Road
London SW3 5EN
Telephone:0171 351 5775

DINOSAUR DESIGNS
Enquiries to:
Level 3/2 Bellevue Street
Surry Hills
Sydney
NSW 2010
Telephone: 02 9211 5353

IKEA
255 North Circular Road
London NW10 OJQ
Telephone 0181 233 2300

GALLERY OF ANTIQUE
COSTUME & TEXTILES
2 Church Street
Marylebone
London NW8 8ED
Telephone: 0171 723 9981

MAPPIN & WEBB
170 Regent Street
London W1R 6BQ
Telephone: 0171 734 3801

JOANNA BOOTH
247 Kings Road
London SW3 5EL
Telephone: 0171 352 8998

PETER CRISP
The Crisp Galleries
"Gap Range"
Bowning
NSW 2582
Telephone: 06 9227 6073
(available at Asprey UK,
Barneys NY)

LINDSAY DAVY
Jeweller and silversmith
19 Commercial Road
Leichhardt
Sydney, NSW 2040
Telephone: 02 9810 3311

COUNTRY ROAD
HOMEWARE
80 - 110 Trenerry Crescent
Collingwood 3066
Victoria, Australia
Telephone: 03 9282 1400

JOSIAH WEDGWOOD
& SONS LTD
BarlastonÈ
Stoke-on-Trent
Staffordshire
Telephone: 01782 204 141

LALIQUE
182 New Bond Street
London W1Y 9PA
Telephone: 0171 499 8228

MINTON
London Road
Stoke on Trent
Staffordshire
ST4 7QP
Tel: 01782 292 292

UNITED CUTLERS
OF SHEFFIELD
Petre Street
Sheffield S4 8LL
Tel: 0114 2433984

ASPREY
(BOND STREET) LTD
165-169 New Bond Street
London W1Y OAR
Telephone: 0171 493 6767

RICARD GINORI
CHINA FROM ICTC
3 Caley Close
Sweet Briar Road
Norwich NR3 2BU
Telephone: 01603 488019

LUNN ANTIQUES
86 New King's Road
London SW6 4LU
Telephone: 0171 736 4638

STUART CRYSTAL
Redhouse Glassworks
Stourbridge
West Midland, DY8 4AA
Telephone: 01384 828282

GARRARD & CO LTD.
Crown Jewellers
112 Regent Street
London W1
Telephone: 0171 734 7020

ACKNOWLEDGEMENTS

I wish to warmly thank everyone who has helped and encouraged me with this book including friends, past colleagues, china companies and stores who lent me their precious merchandise to photograph – especially Maryse and Bob Boxer at Chez Joseph, Thomas Goode, Janet Kennedy for Spode, Wedgwood, everybody at Dinosaur Designs, Sharyn Storrier Lyneham and Vogue Entertaining for inspiration, Peter Crisp, Lindsay Davy and The Beach Road Restaurant, Palm Beach, Sydney for letting me use their premises as a location.

I particularly wish to thank my brilliant assistant Shaun Ford for his hard work, enthusiasm and cheerful company. Malcolm and Eileen Webster who generously let me turn their house into a photographic studio, use all their china, glass and linen and even polished the silver for me. Bertie and Madge Varnham for locking me in a room and making me write the text. Lena Urmossy for her invaluable help with flower arrangements, Rosie Stark for the loan of her 'Asiatic Pheasant' collection, Barney Wan, Sarah Rozen, Peter and Joanna Spencer and finally ... without and but for whom ... Geoff Lung and James Merrell for such wonderful, inspiring photography and their enthusiasm and commitment to the project.

Many thanks, MC

INDEX

alfresco eating 70-83
American formal setting 131
anniversary supper 110-13
Asiatic Pheasant 16-20

balance of height 19, 119
banquet, on shoestring 86-91
baskets 64, 75
black and white 36-41
blue and white 8-27
    accessories 26
    Asiatic Pheasant 16-20
    china 9
    French bistro style 10-15
    Harlequin Blue 22-7
    with pink 16-17
bonbonnières 32
Boxer, Maryse, Rainbow china 28-9, 42-5
breakfast in bed 122-3
buffet lunch 92-7

café style 10-15, 67
cake stands 25, 27, 119
candelabra 37, 51, 100-1
candles 30, 32, 100-1, 104-5, 106, 110-12
chairs, "opera" 86
checks:
    café style 10-15
    gingham 71, 72, 75
China:
    blue and white ware 9
    chopsticks 52-3, 54, 55
Chinese style 52-5
    formal setting 134
chopsticks 52-3, 54, 55
Christmas Day 104-9
coffee pots, brass 57
coffee sets 16, 35, 44, 114-15
contemporary settings 28-49
country settings 14-15
Crisp, Peter, tableware 98-103
crowded tables, settings for 89, 130
cutlery see flatware

Davey, Lyndsey, silverware 98-9
decanters 32, 100-1
Delft ware 9
dinner party 100-1
Dinosaur Designs, frosted resin ware 83
Dresden china 122-3

eggcups 103
English formal setting 129

Fes bowls 56
finger bowls 32
flatware:
    café-style 67
    Chinese 54
    colored-handled 43, 47, 80
    Crisp design 98-9
    crossing 89
    glass-handled 80
    gold-decorated 30-1
    informal setting 13
    plastic-handled 43
    rose-patterned 120, 121, 124-5
    types 136-7
floral pattern 16, 21, 23, 115, 120-5
flowers:
    anemones 72-3
    at place settings 105, 109
    Christmas 104-5, 108-9
    country 12, 15, 26, 64
    daisies 10-11
    gardenias 98, 100-1, 102-3
    Gerber daisies 42-3, 49
    grape hyacinths 122-3
    height of table settings 25
    iris 88
    jasmine 55
    marigolds 64
    peonies 16, 19, 55
    poppies 52, 55
    on plates 25
    ranunculus 122-3
    roses 19, 30-1, 32, 35, 110, 112, 116, 120
        as china pattern 120-1, 124-5
        on flatware 120, 121, 124-5
        on napkin rings 32, 35, 120
        as theme 114-27
    still-life displays 96-7
    sunflowers 64-5
    waterlilies 78-9, 80-1, 82, 83

forks:
    pastry 120, 121
    types 136-7

Fornasetti china 29, 36-7, 39, 40-1
French bistro 10-15
French formal setting 132
fruits 24-5, 32, 45, 49, 61, 95, 96-7

Georgian Plate Collection 22-3
glassware:
    café-style 12
    clear 32
    colored 45, 48-9
    drinking glasses, types 135
    frosted 116
    gold-rimmed 30-1, 36-7
    hand-blown 45, 49
    mint tea glasses 56, 57
    ornamented 98-9
    rose-patterned 124-5
    sorbet colors 83
    wine glasses 23
        for desserts 90
        hock 23
        placement 34-5
        types 135
gold decoration 98-9
gold and silver 102-3, 110-13
gold and white scheme 30-5

Harlequin Blue 22-7
height, balance of 19, 119

Italian formal setting 133

knives:
    blue-handled 22
    types 136-7

lanterns 51
Limoges plates 121
lunch, grand buffet 92-7

Mediterranean style 51, 64-9
mint tea 62-3
    glasses 56, 57, 62-3
    teapot 57, 62-3
Minton Riverton design 112
Moroccan style 51, 56-63
mugs, as vases 86, 90

napkin rings 32, 35, 100-1, 103, 112, 120

napkins:

check 10, 13
    in Chinese setting 55
    Christmas decoration 107
    embroidered 75
    folding 22, 94-5, 124, 138
    gold-bordered 30
    knotted 47
    mismatched 13
    placement 35

perfume shakers 56, 60-1
pewter 95
    creating effect 107
picnic-time 71, 72-7
pitchers 14, 15, 72, 76, 86-7, 90
place cards 89, 139

Quartermain, Carolyn, fabric 113
Quimper pottery 66-7

rainbow colors 28-9, 42-9
resin, frosted 78-83
rose water 32, 56, 61
Rowe, Keith, glassware 48-9
Royal Copenhagen china 9, 27
rustic tableware 67, 69

Safi bowls 56
St Valentine's Day supper 47, 110-13
salad plates 112
salt and pepper sets 12, 31, 37, 80, 100-1
hells, for condiments 72
silver and gold 102-3, 110-13
sorbet colors 78-83
Spode china 9, 22-3, 23
spoons:
    Chinese 54
    French style 100
    types 136-7
Staffordshire pottery 9
still-life displays 92-3, 95, 96-7
suppers:
    candlelit, for two 110-13
    party setting, blue and white 24-5

table linen:
    blue and white 10-15

chenille 95
Chinese pattern 53
damask 95, 104-5
Designers Guild fabric 66-7
embroidered 16, 26
exotic fabrics 51
gingham 71, 72, 75
organdy inset with mirrors 46
organza 116-17
for picnic 72-7
Renaissance Collage 38-9
roses sewn on 118
shantung 52-3, 55
sheets as 86
silk-screened fabric 113
upholstery fabric 36-7, 66-7
table settings:
    American formal 131
    Chinese formal 134
    for crowded table 89, 130
    English formal 129
    French formal 132
    international 129, 131-4
    Italian formal 133
tables:
    refectory 99
    trestle 86
tagine dishes 57
tapestry, Flemish 92-3
tea services:
    Chinese 53
    Victorian 120
tea setting 116-17
teapots:
    Chinese 54
    Moroccan 57
terracotta pottery 64, 66-7, 96
Timney Fowler, linen 38-9
tin dishes 104, 107
toothpicks 61

vases 15, 38-9, 49, 72, 76, 86-7, 90, 96, 105, 109
vegetables, still-life displays 95, 96-7

wedding china 29, 30-31
white, use of 7, 29
wine-cooler, outdoor 72